# Basic Notes in Psychotherapy

14/2/97

To / Giles House

Best wishes,

Mike Levi

**Previous books by the same author**

Levi, M.I. (1987) MCQs for the MRCPsych Part I (Lancaster: MTP Press)

Levi, M.I. (1988) MCQs for the MRCPsych Part II (Lancaster: Kluwer Academic Publishers)

Levi, M.I. (1988) SAQs for the MRCPsych Part II (Lancaster: Kluwer Academic Publishers)

Levi, M.I. (1989) Basic Notes in Psychiatry (Lancaster: Kluwer Academic Publishers). Revised edition 1992

Levi, M.I. (1992) PMPs for the MRCPsych Part II (Lancaster: Kluwer Academic Publishers)

Levi, M.I. (1993) Basic Notes in Psychopharmacology (Lancaster: Kluwer Academic Publishers)

# Basic Notes in Psychotherapy

by

**Dr. Michael I. Levi** MB BS MRCPsych
*Consultant Psychiatrist*
*Lomond Healthcare NHS Trust*
*Vale of Leven District General Hospital*
*Alexandria, Dunbartonshire, Scotland, UK*

**PETROC PRESS**

*Petroc Press,* an imprint of LibraPharm Limited

**Distributors**

Plymbridge Distributors Limited, Plymbridge House, Estover Road, Plymouth PL6 7PZ, UK

**Copyright**

©1996 LibraPharm Limited

All rights reserved. No part of this publication may be reproduced, stored in a retrieval system, or transmitted in any form or by any means, electronic, mechanical, photocopying, recording or otherwise, without prior permission from the publishers.

While every attempt has been made to ensure that the information provided in this book is correct at the time of printing, the publisher, its distributors, sponsors and agents, make no representation, express or otherwise, with regard to the accuracy of the information contained herein and cannot accept any legal responsibility or liability for any errors or omissions that may have been made or for any loss or damage resulting from the use of the information. Lundbeck has expressed no desire for editorial imput into this publication.

Published in the United Kingdom by
LibraPharm Limited, *Gemini House*, 162 Craven Road, Newbury, Berkshire RG14 5NR, UK

A catalogue record for this book is available from the British Library

ISBN 1 900603 50 0

Typeset by
Richard Powell Editorial and Production Services, Basingstoke, Hants
Printed and bound in the United Kingdom by
BPC Wheatons Ltd, Exeter, Devon

# Contents

| | |
|---|---|
| Foreword | 6 |
| Introduction | 7 |
| Acknowledgements | 8 |
| 1. Counselling | 9 |
| 2. Supportive Psychotherapy | 11 |
| 3. Individual Dynamic Psychotherapy | 13 |
| 4. Group Psychotherapy | 22 |
| 5. Couple and Family Therapy | 27 |
| 6. Cognitive Analytical Therapy (CAT) | 31 |
| 7. Cognitive Therapy | 34 |
| 8. Behavioural Therapy | 36 |
| 9. Other Psychotherapies: | |
| (a) Technique in client-centred psychotherapy | 51 |
| (b) Technique in Gestalt therapy | 51 |
| (c) Technique in psychodrama | 52 |
| (d) Technique in transactional analysis | 53 |
| (e) Technique in psychosynthesis | 54 |
| (f) Technique in rational-emotive therapy (RET) | 54 |
| (g) Indications/cautions | 55 |

# Foreword

I well remember as a trainee psychiatrist being thoroughly confused by the myriad of different approaches to providing psychological treatment and the confusion created by obscure jargon handled often in a dogmatic manner, combined with the mutual intolerance sometimes shown by the devotees of different methods. Thankfully, nowadays the experts are beginning to talk about the ways different methods can compliment each other and even become integrated, such as in cognitive analytical and cognitive behavioural therapy.

Dr Levi has managed to distil the key facts from the great complexities of this field of knowledge in such a way that I am sure it will be useful to trainees within any professional group working in mental health. These basic notes will also be an excellent means to introduce medical students and general practitioners to clinically useful psychological concepts, as well as psychiatric trainees at the beginning of their careers. This introduction will, I am sure, set them on a smoother path of understanding than the one on which I started.

Gwyn Davies MB ChB BSc (Hons) MRCPsych
Consultant Psychiatrist
Old Manor Hospital
Salisbury

# Introduction

The purpose of writing this book is to provide a concise summary of psychotherapy in the form of notes.

The psychotherapies discussed in this book are those considered by the author to be the most important psychological treatments that the practising physician needs to know about.

The aim is to provide the principal techniques, indications and cautions of the psychological treatments covered.

I have based these notes on a number of books[1-5]. These notes represent my own view of current clinical practice and are written from the perspective of the general adult psychiatrist.

The book is intended to have wide readership – particularly among junior hospital psychiatrists, general practitioners and medical students. In addition, the book will also be useful to psychiatric nurses, clinical psychologists, psychiatric social workers and psychiatric occupational therapists.

The book attempts to put psychotherapy ('the talking treatments') in straightforward, non-jargon terms. Other books on psychotherapy tend to over-jargon and over-complicate matters; the reader should find that this book is written in an easily understandable way.

## References

1. Bloch S, ed. An Introduction to the Psychotherapies, second edition, 1986: Oxford University Press
2. Brown D, Pedder J. Introduction to Psychotherapy, second edition, 1993: Routledge
3. Holmes J, ed. Textbook of Psychotherapy in Psychiatric Practice, 1991: Churchill Livingstone
4. Kendell RE, Zealley AK, eds. Companion to Psychiatric Studies, fifth edition, 1993: Churchill Livingstone
5. Maxwell H, ed. An Outline of Psychotherapy, second edition, 1991: Whurr Publishers Ltd

# Acknowledgements

The author is indebted to Dr Andrew Clarke for his invaluable help in reviewing the manuscript.

Thanks are also due to Mr Adrian Childs-Clarke and Dr John Hook for their advice and encouragement.

Many thanks also to Dr T. G. Davies for his helpful comments and for providing the Foreword to the book.

# CHAPTER 1

# Counselling

## (a) TECHNIQUE

Counselling can be broken down into the following components:

(i) facilitation of the expression of affect thereby reducing emotional tension.

(ii) reflection, clarification and reassurance thereby enabling the patient to think more clearly about problems.

(iii) facilitation of the patient's understanding of problems.

(iv) facilitation of problem solving so that the patient can find new ways of tackling problems.

## (b) INDICATIONS

(i) To enable people to cope more effectively with the current problems of living, e.g. acute stress reactions – people experiencing acute psychological distress (in response to life events or relationship problems) in the absence of mental illness.

(ii) For most brief anxiety disorders, counselling with an emphasis on reassurance is usually sufficient, i.e. anxiolytic drugs need not be prescribed.

## (c) CAUTION

(i) 'Giving expert advice' – the patient may need advice of a medical, legal or financial nature. It is usually preferable for such advice to come from a specialist agency not involved in the counselling.

*N.B.* The patient's need to take responsibility for decisions and actions should not be undermined.

(ii) Patients with personality disorder, where the problems are too deep seated to be changed by counselling. Here there must be an awareness of the need to refer such patients for more formal psychotherapy.

**CHAPTER 2**

# Supportive Psychotherapy

## (a) TECHNIQUE

Supportive psychotherapy can be broken down into the following components:

(i) Listening – listening carefully to what the patient is saying, picking up verbal and non-verbal clues, and enabling the patient to give a full account of the situation and problems, can result in a significant improvement.

(ii) Reassurance – this can be used to good effect to relieve fears, boost self-confidence and promote hope.

(iii) Explanation – explaining to a patient why they are experiencing certain symptoms can itself be reassuring and therapeutic.

(iv) Guidance and suggestion – advice may be necessary with regard to a particular problem, such as handling a job interview or to general issues, such as making contact with members of the opposite sex.

(v) Expression of feelings – it does seem useful for patients to be able to express emotions such as anger, frustration and despair openly within a supportive setting.

## (b) INDICATION

Relevant to all forms of psychiatric disorder and part of good general psychiatric practice; the supportive relationship any member of the multidisciplinary team has with a patient; the primary aim is to maintain their functioning capacity, maintain their defences and strengths and help promote their adaptation to everyday living.

## (c) CAUTION

The problem of dependence – the therapist does not want to encourage the patient's dependence on himself/herself. If it occurs, when therapy is withdrawn, the patient will not be able to cope.

# CHAPTER 3

# Individual Dynamic Psychotherapy

## (a) BASIC CONCEPTS

### (i) Introduction

1. Individual dynamic psychotherapy is based on the premise that a person's behaviour is influenced by unconscious factors.

2. The unconscious refers to a combination of thoughts, feelings and fantasies of which we are unaware, and which influence our behaviour.

### (ii) Evidence for the existence of unconscious activity:

This comes from a variety of sources:

1. Dreams – in which the manifest (overt) content of dreams is interpreted in terms of the latent (hidden) content of dreams, i.e. the deeper meaning.

2. Artistic and scientific creativity – many artists and scientists, in describing their own creative processes, have told of how they feel taken over by some inner force, not entirely within their conscious control.

3. Hysterical symptoms – according to psychoanalytical theory, hysterics suffer from the effects of emotionally charged ideas lodged in the unconscious at some

time in the past. Symptoms are explained as the combined effects of repression and the 'conversion' of emotional energy into physical channels.

4. Abreaction – this used to be part of the management of hysteria brought about by a slow intravenous injection of ten milligrams of diazepam. In the resulting state, the patient was encouraged to relive the stressful events that provoked the hysterical symptoms and to express the accompanying emotions.

5. Parapraxes – apparent omissions or errors occurring in everyday life ('slips of the tongue') which are symbolic of underlying attitudes.

### (iii) Psychological defence mechanisms:

1. These are strategies used by the unconscious mind to keep out unconscious material in order to cope with the realities of everyday life. They help to reduce anxiety.

2. The most important defence mechanisms are:

   (A) Denial – the refusal to recognise external reality.
   (B) Isolation – the isolation of thoughts or behaviour so that their links with other thoughts or with the rest of the patient's life are broken.
   (C) Projection – the attribution of one's own unacknowledged feelings to others.
   (D) Reaction formation – the development of a feeling which is opposite to that really present.
   (E) Regression – the return to an earlier stage of psychological development.

- (F) Repression – the basic psychological defence mechanism whereby anxiety-provoking thoughts are pushed into the unconscious.
- (G) Sublimation – the diversion of one's unacceptable feelings into more socially acceptable activities.
- (H) Turning on the self – the process whereby unacceptable aggression towards others is directed towards one's self.
- (I) Displacement – the redirection of emotions from one object to another.

### (iv) Transference and Counter-transference:

1. Transference is defined as those feelings the patient has towards the therapist which are reminiscent of the patient's feelings towards significant persons during his/her development.

2. Counter-transference is defined as those feelings the therapist has towards the patient which are reminiscent of the therapist's feelings towards significant persons during his/her development and are evoked by the patient.

## (b) TECHNIQUE

(i) The distinctive feature of individual dynamic psychotherapy is its focus on those unconscious mental processes which are thought to underlie the patient's symptoms or presenting problem.

(ii) The therapeutic relationship (therapeutic alliance) is regarded as the critical element in individual dynamic psychotherapy because it is in the context of this safe, caring but professional relationship that the patient can become aware of, and explore, the significance of this unconscious material.

(iii) The patient will be helped to understand feelings and patterns of relating to others. The patterns will be explored through transference to the therapist and will be linked with significant relationships and events in the patient's life.

(iv) The therapist will use his/her countertransference to give clues as to the patient's non-verbalised feelings.

(v) A certain amount of personal therapy for the therapist may be necessary in order to enable him/her to distinguish between his/her own problems and those of the patient.

(vi) Individual dynamic psychotherapy may be either brief (short-term) or long-term:

1. In brief psychotherapy the therapist is usually more active, whereas in long-term psychotherapy the therapist is usually more reflective.

2. Brief psychotherapy refers to weekly treatment for a maximum of six months, whereas long-term psychotherapy refers to treatment at least once a week for at least nine months.

3. Most of the individual dynamic psychotherapy available in the National Health Service is brief psychotherapy. Only a relatively small proportion of attenders at psychotherapy departments have long-term psychotherapy, although it is on

# INDIVIDUAL DYNAMIC PSYCHOTHERAPY

this group that the majority of professional resources are concentrated.

(vii) In summary, individual dynamic psychotherapy is intended to effect change in the patient by:

1. Confrontation of the patient's psychological defence mechanisms.

2. Clarification and understanding of the patient's problems.

3. Interpretation of the patient's unconscious material permitting new formulations of previous problems.

# (c) GENERAL INDICATIONS

(i) Psychological understandability – the patient's difficulties must be understandable in psychological terms.

(ii) Psychological mindedness – the patient's capacity to think about his problems in psychological terms.

(iii) Motivation – the patient must have sufficient motivation for insight and change.

(iv) Intelligence and verbal fluency – average intelligence and verbal fluency are desirable, otherwise the patient's capacity to communicate through talking may be restricted.

(v) Introspectiveness – a degree of introspectiveness is desirable, otherwise patients will find it difficult to reflect and think about their feelings.

(vi) Dreams – the capacity to remember dreams is another useful indicator of the ability of patients to contact unconscious parts of themselves.

(vii) Ego strength – the patient must have adequate ego strength, which includes the capacity to tolerate frustrating or disturbing feelings without engaging in impulsive behaviour.

(viii) Capacity to form relationships – the patient must have the capacity to form and sustain relationships; even one sustained relationship in the patient's past or current life suggests a firmer basis from which to start psychotherapy.

# (d) SPECIFIC INDICATIONS

Patients with:

(i) Relationship problems.

(ii) Grief reactions.

(iii) Psychosomatic disorders.

(iv) Personality difficulties – that is personality traits which cause distress, but which do not amount to a personality disorder.

(v) Personality disorders.

(vi) Hysteria.

(vii) Generalised anxiety disorders.

(viii) Depressive disorders – most clinicians restrict the use of individual dynamic psychotherapy to less severe depressive disorders. Occasionally those with severe depressive disorders which have been medically stabilised can be treated with individual dynamic psychotherapy.

(ix) 'Transitional crises' (e.g. leaving home, marriage, parenthood, retirement) – such patients are often excellent candidates for brief psychotherapy.

*N.B.* Brief psychotherapy in general is only likely to be helpful when most of the patient's difficulties revolve around a core conflict that can be defined in psychodynamic terms and serve as a focus for therapy.

# (e) GENERAL CAUTIONS

(i) Repeated hospital admissions, frequent suicidal attempts, repeated risk taking or serious somatisation into major psychosomatic disorder, may suggest insufficient ego strength for psychotherapy.

(ii) A history of repeated dropping-out of relationships or repeated failures to complete ventures are bad predictors for sticking at psychotherapy.

(iii) In general, patients with acute psychotic disorders are not amenable to psychotherapy.

(iv) Severely depressed patients may be too slowed up and unresponsive to psychotherapy.

- (v) There may be a need to combine psychotropic drugs with psychotherapy. Over-sedation should be avoided as this may hinder the patient's capacity to access feelings.

- (vi) Patients who are actively abusing alcohol or illicit drugs are not amenable to psychotherapy.

- (vii) Very limited intelligence and verbal fluency.

- (viii) No real motivation to change or grossly unreal expectations of individual dynamic psychotherapy.

- (ix) A lack of personal, social and family resources to cope with the demands of individual dynamic psychotherapy.

## (f) SPECIFIC CAUTIONS (some overlap with general cautions)

Individual dynamic psychotherapy should not be used in patients with:

- (i) Risk of overdependence in one to one therapy.

- (ii) Risk of personality clash with the therapist.

- (iii) Very limited intelligence and verbal fluency.

- (iv) No real motivation to change or grossly unreal expectations of psychodynamic psychotherapy.

- (v) A lack of personal, social and family resources to cope with the demands of psychodynamic psychotherapy.

(vi) A difficulty in thinking in psychological terms, who are not introspective, and who are unable to reflect frankly on themselves.

# CHAPTER 4

# Group Psychotherapy

## (a) TECHNIQUE

(i) In group psychotherapy the main therapeutic agent is the group itself.

(ii) The group psychotherapist requires training in the recognition and utilisation of the following specific group events:

1. Socialisation – the learning from others through acceptance and inclusion.

2. Mirror phenomena – the patient seeing aspects of himself reflected in fellow patients.

3. Commonality – obscure meanings become more evident through being pooled.

4. Sharing – contagion of emotions such as rage and grief when the patient is moved to experience emotions which fellow patients express.

(iii) There are two types of group:

1. Closed groups – these run for a fixed period of time with the same members (the optimal number of patients being eight). New members do not join during the course of the group.

2. Open groups – these usually have no fixed time

period and do take in new members as others leave.

(iv) Group process:

1. There is no formal agenda for group discussion and the therapist will not initially offer any direction, leaving the other members of the group to talk about anything they want to bring up.

2. The therapist will allow this process to develop, watching and listening, and will then contribute to the group discussion to enable the group members to learn from their own experience of participating in the group process.

(v) The following are recognised to be key therapeutic factors in group therapy:

1. Interpersonal learning – learning from one's constructive and adaptive relationship with others.

2. Catharsis – the experience of relief through expression of feelings.

3. Group cohesiveness – the sense that one is valued and belongs to the group.

4. Insight/self-understanding – the generation of self-awareness and understanding of one's actions and motives.

5. Development of socialising techniques.

6. Universality – the recognition that one's

problems are not unique.

7. Instillation of hope – seeing other members of the group making positive changes can instil hope.

8. Altruism – the experience of being helpful and of value to others.

9. Vicarious learning – learning about oneself through the observation of other group members, including the therapist.

10. Guidance – the receipt of advice or information.

# (b) GENERAL INDICATIONS

*See* Individual Dynamic Psychotherapy

# (c) SPECIFIC INDICATIONS

(i) Personality disorders (in general) – group psychotherapy is usually more helpful than individual psychotherapy.

(ii) Antisocial personality disorders – people with antisocial personality disorders are usually resistant to psychotherapy, although some are helped by large group psychotherapy in the form of a therapeutic community. In such a unit, the patients meet several times a day for group discussions, in which each person's behaviour and feelings are examined by the other group members.

# GROUP PSYCHOTHERAPY

(iii) Alcohol and drug dependence:

1. Group psychotherapy is used to help patients develop insight into their emotional and personality problems.

2. Group psychotherapy aims to enable patients to observe their own problems mirrored in other substance abusers and to work out better ways of coping with their problems.

3. Group psychotherapy is the most widely used intensive treatment for substance abusers.
*N.B.* Group psychotherapy will not be helpful whilst the patient is still actively abusing alcohol or illicit drugs.

(iv) Victims of childhood sexual abuse – it is often helpful for victims to share their experiences and their feelings of guilt, shame, anger and disgust with each other.

(v) People with difficulties in socialisation – group psychotherapy may offer them an opportunity to learn how to interact with other people.

## (d) GENERAL CAUTIONS

*See* Individual Dynamic Psychotherapy

## (e) SPECIFIC CAUTIONS

Group psychotherapy should not be used in patients:

(i) Who definitely do not want to participate in a group.

(ii) With a lack of impulse control such that the safety of other group members is at risk.

(iii) With an immediate crisis requiring immediate help, with no time to enter a group and establish relationships that can lead to change.

(iv) With a speech impediment or other language difficulty sufficient to inhibit ordinary conversation.

(v) Who would be at high risk of being an outcast in a group.

# CHAPTER 5

# Couple and Family Therapy

## (a) TECHNIQUE

There are three models which are generally used in couple and family therapy:

(i) The psychodynamic model – this model is concerned with:

1. The intrapsychic life of the individual members of the couple or family.

2. The influence of past, personal and family histories on present relationships and functioning.

3. The use of reflection and interpretation as a means of generating insight and hence mobilising change in relationships and behaviour.

4. The recognition of transference phenomena as a way of understanding relationships and working through problems in them.

(ii) The behavioural model – this model seeks to define those behaviours which:

1. Are dysfunctional for the people concerned.

2. Can be altered by the setting of appropriate goals and tasks to achieve them.

3. Can be regularly monitored, reviewed and evaluated.

*N.B.* It is important that the tasks that are set by the therapist are specific and agreeable to the individuals involved.

(iii) The systemic model – this model sees the couple or family as a dynamic system where problems between individual members are viewed as a reflection of problems in the system as a whole. Working with the model, the therapist:

1. Seeks to modify the change-resisting dynamics of couple or family relationships.

2. Helps the couple or family to rewrite their 'script', and redefine their roles by exploring and testing out new possibilities of relating to each other.

# (b) SELECTION CRITERIA

(i) Agreement by the couple or family that there is a problem requiring resolution.

(ii) A willingness of the couple or family to commit themselves to attend sessions.

(iii) The likelihood that the couple or family will remain together throughout the planned course of work.

(iv) When the problem is evidence of one or more

individuals struggling for differentiation and independence.

(v) When the problem is evidence of one or more individuals struggling to avoid being caught up or enmeshed in the disturbance of others.

(vi) When one spouse or family member is the carrier of, reactor against, or scapegoat for, serious unrecognised problems in other members of the family, or colludes with such disturbance to their mutual disadvantage.

(vii) When there is a grossly disturbed family member who resists individual work but who might accept help when shared by the spouse or family.

# (c) INDICATIONS

(i) Relationship difficulties

(ii) Depressive disorders – couple or family therapy aims to alleviate the problems that led to the disorder in the identified patient.

(iii) Schizophrenia – family therapy may be beneficial to families, especially when directed at reducing their expressed emotion.

(iv) Anorexia nervosa – family therapy has been advocated since problems in family relationships are common in anorexia nervosa.
*N.B.* **Family therapy is particularly useful in child psychiatric disorders.**

## (d) CAUTIONS

Couple and family therapy should not be used in:

(i) Couples and families which are very close to separation.

(ii) Couples and families who, despite their sincere pleas for help, are so entrenched in their relationships, that their commitment to making use of help is accompanied by a firm need to resist change.

# CHAPTER 6
# Cognitive Analytical Therapy (CAT)

## (a) TECHNIQUE

(i) CAT is a brief, time-limited therapy usually lasting twenty sessions.

(ii) Its theoretical base draws upon both cognitive and psychoanalytical sources – the attempt has been made to restate key psychoanalytic concepts in a language compatible with current thinking in cognitive theory.

(iii) The central task of CAT is to help the patient revise patterns of thought, feeling and behaviour which were adaptive in a traumatic early life but which cause problems in adult life.

(iv) At the beginning of treatment, the patient is given a rationale of the treatment, 'the psychotherapy file'. This removes some of the mystery of the therapeutic process, by describing the current patterns of habitual distorted thinking, as well as explaining their origins in the emotional conflict endured in childhood.

(v) The basis of treatment is the 'CAT reformulation', undertaken as a joint task by the patient and the therapist, and written down or represented diagrammatically.

(vi) Target problems and the procedures which maintain

these problems are identified and tackled during therapy.

(vii) The ending of therapy is formally addressed through the exchange of 'goodbye letters' between patient and therapist, in which the progress through therapy is reviewed and any difficulties about ending are explicitly discussed.

(viii) CAT considers that most distortions of thinking can be classified within three groups:

1. Traps – patterns of thinking and behaving which are 'vicious circles', so that in trying to deal with bad feelings, the resulting thinking or action tends to confirm the badness.

2. Snags – the internal and external limitations experienced by the patient as making change impossible. Either people around the patient prefer him not to change, or the patient himself somehow seems to 'arrange' to avoid pleasure or success.

3. Dilemmas – where thinking is polarised into false choices or either/or options.

# (b) INDICATIONS

(i) Abnormal grief reactions.

(ii) Depressive and anxiety disorders.

(iii) Most personality disorders (including the borderline type) – with more experienced therapists these patients, who may be unsuitable for individual dynamic psychotherapy, can make impressive gains with this treatment.

# CHAPTER 7

# Cognitive Therapy

## (a) TECHNIQUE

(i) Beck suggests that a person who habitually adopts ways of thinking with depressed or anxious 'cognitive distortions', will be more likely to become depressed or anxious when faced with minor problems.

(ii) There are four basic types of error shown by 'cognitive distortions' in cognitive theory:

1. Arbitrary inference – drawing a conclusion when there is no evidence for it and even some against it.

2. Selective abstraction – focusing on a detail and ignoring more important features of a situation.

3. Over-generalisation – drawing a general conclusion on the basis of a single incident.

4. Minimisation and magnification – performance is underestimated and errors are overestimated.

(iii) These mechanisms lead to distortions within the cognitive triad of:

1. Evaluation of the self.

2. View of life experiences.

3. View of the future.

(iv) In cognitive therapy, the patient first learns to identify 'cognitive distortions' from present or recent experiences with the use of daily records (Beck's diaries).

(v) The patient records such ideas and then learns to examine the evidence for and against them, i.e. tests out beliefs in real life.

(vi) The patient can be encouraged to undertake some of the pleasurable activities that were given up at the onset of depression or anxiety.

(vii) In this way, the patient attempts 'cognitive restructuring', i.e. he/she attempts to identify, evaluate and change his/her distorted thoughts and associated behaviours.

# (b) INDICATIONS

(i) Depressive disorders (synergistic with antidepressant drug therapy).

(ii) Anxiety disorders (generalised anxiety disorder and panic disorder).

(iii) Increasingly cognitive therapy has been adapted to undertake more in-depth problems, e.g. victims of sexual abuse.

(iv) Eating disorders.

(v) Hypochondriasis.

**CHAPTER 8**

# Behavioural Therapy

## 1. RELAXATION TRAINING

### (a) TECHNIQUE

Relaxation training can take several forms:

(i) A procedure using a simple system of exercises intended to bring about progressive relaxation of individual groups of skeletal muscles and to regulate breathing.

(ii) A procedure using a simple system of taped instructions intended to bring about relaxation – it is usual to link the resulting relaxed state with a pleasant, imagined scene so that relaxation can be induced in any situation merely by recalling the imagined scene.

### (b) INDICATIONS

(i) Such simple relaxation is effective in reducing mild to moderate anxiety, but not severe anxiety.

(ii) Relaxation training is useful in the management of phobias and panic disorder, as long as it is combined with exposure tasks and the patient is taught how to apply it.

## 2. ANXIETY MANAGEMENT TRAINING (AMT)

### (a) TECHNIQUE

This procedure involves two stages:

   (i) Verbal cues and mental imagery are used to arouse anxiety.

   (ii) The patient is trained to reduce this anxiety by relaxation, distraction and reassuring self-statements.

### (b) INDICATIONS

AMT may be more effective in reducing anxiety than simple relaxation training, especially if the positive self-statements are individualised and address the patient's specific fear-evoking cognitions.


## 3. SYSTEMATIC DESENSITISATION (SD) IN IMAGINATION

### (a) TECHNIQUE

   (i) Patients are required to imagine the anxiety-provoking objects or situation vividly, starting with those that evoke little fear and progressing through carefully planned stages (a 'hierarchy') until the patient habituates, i.e. becomes accustomed to the anxiety by frequent exposure, and the avoidance response is extinguished.

(ii) At each stage, anxiety is neutralised by relaxation training (*see* Relaxation Training at the beginning of this chapter).

### (b) INDICATION

Effective in the treatment of simple phobic disorders of an object or situation not encountered readily (e.g. aeroplanes).

## 4. EXPOSURE *IN VIVO*

### (a) TECHNIQUE

(i) Patients are exposed to the cues of triggers of anxiety-provoking objects or situations, with a similar progression up the 'hierarchy' as described in Systematic Desensitisation In Imagination, using real life situations in a graded manner of exposure.

(ii) Habituation can be enhanced by simple anxiety management techniques.

### (b) INDICATIONS

(i) Effective in the treatment of simple phobic neuroses of an object or situation encountered readily.

(ii) Effective in the treatment of agoraphobia, when it is combined with training patients to overcome avoidance behaviour in a planned way, the practice of which is carried out each day. This total package of treatment is known as programmed practice and is the treatment of choice in agoraphobia.
*N.B.* In agoraphobia, the spouse can often be usefully used as a co-therapist.

# 5. FLOODING/IMPLOSION

## (a) TECHNIQUE

(i) Flooding involves prolonged exposure of patients *in vivo* to phobic objects or situations in a non-graded manner with a view to promote extinction of anxiety.

(ii) Implosion involves exposing patients in imagination to phobic objects or situations in a non-graded manner with no attempt to reduce anxiety. Invariably, patients are taken over and above the top item of the hierarchy, e.g. spiders crawling all over the body, *cf.* flooding, where patients are taken to the top item of the hierarchy, e.g. spiders crawling on the hand.
*N.B.* Both flooding and implosion involve a maximum exposure of patients to anxiety-provoking objects or situations, i.e. exposing patients to items at the top of the hierarchy (flooding) or items over and above the top of the hierarchy (implosion).

## (b) INDICATIONS

(i) This behavioural therapy is as effective as Systematic Desensitisation (SD) In Imagination in the treatment of phobias – generally the decision whether to use this therapy or SD In Imagination will be by the mutual agreement of the patient and the therapist; the effect of treatment is usually much quicker with this treatment, *cf.* SD In Imagination, but the phobic response tends to build up again between sessions with flooding/implosion, with a steady reduction in fear in succeeding sessions.

(ii) Flooding is more effective, *cf.* SD in imagination in the treatment of obsessive compulsive disorders when combined with response prevention (see later section).

(iii) This therapy is particularly effective in patients with free-floating anxiety.

# 6. RESPONSE PREVENTION

## (a) TECHNIQUE

(i) Response prevention can be used in combination with flooding (see earlier section) or in a graded way.

(ii) The technique involves exposing the patient to a contaminating object such as a toilet seat or a soiled towel, i.e. exposing the patient to those situations previously evoking compulsive rituals (flooding).

(iii) The patient is subsequently prevented from carrying out the usual compulsive cleansing rituals until the urge to do so has passed (response prevention).

## (b) INDICATIONS

(i) The combination of flooding and response prevention is the behavioural treatment of choice in the treatment of obsessional thoughts occurring with compulsive rituals – with persistence, the compulsive rituals and the distress subsequently diminish.

(ii) The obsessional thoughts accompanying the rituals usually improve as well with this treatment.

## 7. THOUGHT STOPPING

### (a) TECHNIQUE

(i) The patient is asked to ruminate and, upon doing so, the therapist immediately shouts 'stop' to teach the patient to interrupt the intrusive, obsessional thoughts.

(ii) After considerable practice the patient learns to internalise the 'stop' order so that the thought stopping technique can be used outside the therapy situation.

(iii) Alternatively, the patient can arrest the obsessional thoughts by arranging a sudden intrusion, such as snapping an elastic band on the wrist.

### (b) INDICATION

(i) Thought stopping is indicated in the treatment of obsessional ruminative thoughts occurring without compulsive rituals.

(ii) Thought stopping is also used in the treatment of sexually deviant thoughts.


## 8. THOUGHT SATIATION

### (a) TECHNIQUE

(i) The patient is required deliberately to form the unwanted obsessional ruminative thoughts and retain them for long periods.

(ii) At the same time, the patient is required to refrain from 'neutralising' activities.

(iii) Thus, the patient is instructed to practice forming the unwanted thoughts until tiring of them. This involves the use of tape loops and tape recorders.

(iv) Intolerance of the procedure can be supplemented with progressive muscular relaxation – this is called habituation training.

*N.B.* There is a need to keep changing the thoughts, or they lose their potency.

**(b) INDICATION**

Thought satiation is indicated in the treatment of obsessional ruminations occurring without compulsive rituals.

# 9. SOCIAL SKILLS TRAINING

**(a) TECHNIQUE**

(i) Social skills training aims to modify a patient's social behaviour in order to help overcome difficulties in forming and/or maintaining relationships with other people; in addition to improving social competence, it may also improve the subject's overall psychological adjustment.

(ii) The procedure is applied to patients with social deficits consequent upon psychiatric disorder.

(iii) Video recordings can be used to define and rate elements of the patient's behaviour in standard social encounters.

(iv) The patient is then taught more appropriate behaviour by a combination of direct instruction, modelling, video-feedback and role reversal.

## (b) INDICATIONS

(i) Patients with gross and incapacitating interpersonal difficulties who are not psychotic.

(ii) Patients with problems with assertion.

(iii) Patients with long-term psychiatric disorders as part of a rehabilitation programme – particularly patients with chronic schizophrenia.

(iv) Patients with alcohol abuse – to train them how to refuse a drink.

# 10. TOKEN ECONOMY (POSITIVE REINFORCEMENT)

## (a) TECHNIQUE

(i) This system uses positive and negative reinforcement to alter behaviour.

(ii) Behaviours necessary for effective independent living are specified.

(iii) A unit of exchange (the token) is specified and its presentation to a patient is made contingent upon the occurrence of the required behaviour, i.e. if the patient produces the required behaviour, he receives a number of tokens (positive reinforcement); if the patient fails to produce the required behaviour, the tokens are withheld (negative reinforcement). Thus, the patient benefits or suffers from the consequences of his/her own actions.

(iv) The whole purpose of the token economy regime is to reward patients for behaving appropriately, *cf.* punishing patients for not behaving appropriately. If the programme is too difficult, it should be re-scheduled. The whole point of the regime is lost if it becomes punitive.

(v) It is usual to give tokens that can be used to purchase goods or privileges. Thus, an exchange system is devised, by which a specified number of tokens is required to purchase goods or privileges.

(vi) The aims of the token economy system are:

1. To establish the skills necessary for independent living in the community.

2. To eliminate unwanted behaviours that constitute major management problems for the subject.

3. To improve the subject's overall quality of life.

## (b) INDICATIONS

(i) Patients with long-term psychiatric disorders as part of a rehabilitation programme – particularly patients with chronic schizophrenia.

(ii) Patients with mental handicap.

(iii) Patients with alcohol and drug abuse.

*N.B.* The token economy system has been criticised on ethical grounds with respect to the withholding of goods or privileges from a patient if he/she fails to produce the required behaviour. One way round this difficulty is only to use goods or privileges which are regarded as beyond the basic needs of the patient and are seen as more of a luxury, e.g. additional cigarettes given to the patient over and above the usual number.

# 11. AVERSION THERAPY

## (a) TECHNIQUE

(i) Aversion therapy involves producing an unpleasant sensation in the patient in association with an aversive or noxious stimulus, with the aim of eliminating unwanted behaviours.

(ii) Aversive stimuli include electric shocks, chemically induced nausea and the infliction of pain.

## (b) INDICATIONS

(i) Alcohol dependence syndrome (disulfiram being the aversive stimulus, inducing nausea in the patient if alcohol is consumed).

(ii) Sexual deviations (including patients who sexually abuse children).

(iii) Self-injuring patients.

## (c) CAUTIONS

(i) Aversion therapy has been strongly criticised on ethical grounds, as it sometimes involves inflicting pain on patients.

(ii) Aversion therapy has been commonly used in the past, but has lost popularity nowadays because the results of treatment were rather disappointing.

(iii) In some instances, particularly in the mentally handicapped, aversion therapy can paradoxically increase the undesirable behaviour, thus causing emotional conflict in the patient, and result in aggression towards the therapist.

(iv) Punishment procedures are generally ineffective, unless patients are taught more appropriate behaviours.

# 12. COVERT SENSITISATION

## (a) TECHNIQUE

(i) Covert sensitisation involves the use of aversive stimuli in imagination.

(ii) The technique involves the patient being encouraged to imagine himself/herself performing the unwanted behaviour and then to interrupt this fantasy by simultaneously imagining an aversive or highly unpleasant experience, e.g. the approach of a policeman to arrest him/her for his/her undesirable behaviour.

*N.B.* There is a need to keep changing the scenes, or they lose their potency.

## (b) INDICATIONS

The indications for covert sensitisation are the same as those for aversion therapy (see earlier).

# 13. MODELLING AND ROLE PLAY

## (a) TECHNIQUE

   (i) This refers to the acquisition of new behaviours by the process of imitation.

   (ii) The patient observes the therapist carrying out the required behaviour which the patient finds difficult to perform and then imitates the therapist.

## (b) INDICATIONS

   (i) Phobic disorders.

   (ii) Obsessive compulsive disorders.

   (iii) To develop social skills.

   (iv) To increase self-assertiveness.

# 14. SELF-MONITORING

## (a) TECHNIQUE

   (i) This technique tackles, for example, the hair pulling behaviour in patients with trichotillomania, *cf.* the underlying psychological problems.

(ii) Self-monitoring is a simple approach which involves getting the patient to keep a strict daily log of hair pulling.

(iii) It is often effective.

## (b) INDICATIONS

(i) Habit disorders, e.g. trichotillomania (hair pulling).

(ii) Alcohol and nicotine dependence.

(iii) Depressive and anxiety disorders.

## (c) CAUTION

Self-monitoring makes obsessional patients worse, by increasing awareness of their problems and subsequently increasing compulsivity.

# 15. BIOFEEDBACK

## (a) TECHNIQUE

(i) This technique consists of providing the patient with information about the state of his/her physiological functioning by the use of electronic instruments.

(ii) The most widely used instrument measures the galvanic skin response (GSR), which is a sensitive index of the state of arousal.

(iii) The GSR, or another physiological accompaniment of anxiety such as the heart rate, is electronically converted by the instrument into a visual or auditory signal for the patient.

(iv) The patient learns to alter the signal and thus his/her state of arousal.

## (b) INDICATIONS

(i) Generalised anxiety disorders.

(ii) Tension headaches.

(iii) Migraine.

(iv) Neuromuscular disorders (with the use of electromyographic feedback).

# 16. BELL AND PAD TECHNIQUE

## (a) TECHNIQUE

(i) The patient sleeps on a special pad which completes an electric circuit when it is wetted by urine.

(ii) This causes a bell to ring, which in turn causes the patient to awake and interrupts urination.

(iii) The patient gets up, completes urination and remakes his bed.

(iv) The alarm is reset before the patient goes back to sleep.

## (b) INDICATION

Nocturnal enuresis, especially in children.

# CHAPTER 9

# Other Psychotherapies

## (a) TECHNIQUE IN CLIENT-CENTRED PSYCHOTHERAPY

### Founded by Carl Rogers

Three attitudes of the therapist are deemed to be most important for the success of client-centred psychotherapy:

(i) Genuineness – this means that the therapist is being himself/herself, not denying himself/herself.

(ii) Unconditional positive regard – this refers to the therapist's complete acceptance of his/her client.

(iii) Empathy – this refers to the therapist's ability to enter into the private, inner world of the client, *cf.* merely understanding what he/she is saying.

## (b) TECHNIQUE IN GESTALT THERAPY

### Popularised by Fritz Perls

The important concepts in this therapy are:

(i) The emphasis on valuing experience in the here-and-now.

(ii) To help to expand the patient's self-awareness and to improve his/her relationship with the outside world, so that he/she experiences himself/herself as an organised whole ('Gestalt').

# (c) TECHNIQUE IN PSYCHODRAMA

## *Described by Jacob Moreno*

The important concepts in this therapy are:

(i) The psychodrama session is made up of the therapist, the central subject (patient), other 'players', the audience and the stage.

(ii) The central subject is the group member who becomes the focus of the session and whose life provides the situations which are re-enacted.

(iii) The other 'players' are the other group members who play roles in the central subject's life.

(iv) The audience are professional workers, patients or the central subject's family.

(v) An incident is chosen and the central subject takes centre stage; such re-enacting may include role reversal or role substitution for the patient and the use of props.

# (d) TECHNIQUE IN TRANSACTIONAL ANALYSIS

*Founded by Eric Berne*

The important concepts in this therapy are:

(i) The personality consists of parent, adult and child ego states, i.e. sometimes people behave like parents, sometimes like adults, and sometimes like children.

(ii) Life problems are caused by a lack of appropriateness (congruence) between the respective ego states of participants in interactions, e.g. an adult-child relationship when the appropriate relationship is adult-adult.

(iii) In therapy, the aim is to make the adult ego state stronger by displacing the child and parent ego states from inappropriate situations – this is achieved by exploring the ego defence mechanisms employed by the patient to justify his use of the child and parent ego states as adult states.

(iv) People seek positive strokes (loving, supportive statements) but will settle for negative strokes (hateful, critical statements) if they cannot obtain positive strokes in preference to no strokes at all; in order to obtain the desired number of strokes, people engage in 'games' (repetitive and recurrent patterns of behaviour).

(v) In therapy, the therapist explores with the patient the 'games' which he/she plays with others.

# (e) TECHNIQUE IN PSYCHO-SYNTHESIS

### *Derived from the work of Roberto Assagioli*

The important concepts in this therapy are:

(i) The personality consists of a series of subpersonalities between which a person may shuttle according to the perceived need of the moment.

(ii) Therapy is directed at the recognition and integration of these different subpersonalities into a coherent whole, using a mixture of conversational and dramatic methods.

# (f) TECHNIQUE IN RATIONAL–EMOTIVE THERAPY (RET)

### *Developed by Albert Ellis*

The important concepts in this therapy are:

(i) RET holds that 'neurotic' behaviour derives from one of a number of irrational beliefs which put impossible demands on people.

(ii) Therapy is directed at the recognition and modification of these irrational beliefs in quite a challenging style.

(iii) The basis of treatment is the 'RET reformulation', undertaken as a joint task by the patient and the therapist, and written down.

## (g) INDICATIONS/CAUTIONS

(i) These psychotherapies shift away from the concepts of treatment and cure to notions of self-growth, increased awareness and transformation ('growth therapies', 'human potential movement').

(ii) They also move away from the traditional notion of knowledge and expertise solely residing in the therapist, towards a belief in the therapeutic power of the patient's creativity.

(iii) They tend to attract enthusiastic support, but their emphasis on experience, rather than thinking, can promote a culture in which 'anything goes'.

(iv) They need to be used with discretion and their value with patients with more severe neurotic disorders is questionable.

(v) They are particularly useful in patients who have difficulties in expressing their feelings verbally, e.g. patients with learning difficulties.